KU-720-179

Contents

Acknowledgements

This project was funded by the Joseph Rowntree Foundation. We are grateful to Professor Sally Baldwin, Director of the Social Policy Research Unit, for the provision of additional financial support to fund the evaluation of the key worker service. Many thanks go to the research advisory group for their interest and attendance at the many meetings held during the course of the project.

This project would not have been possible without the sustained commitment and considerable enthusiasm of managers and practitioners from Middlesbrough and North East Lincolnshire who formed the project steering groups. We would also like to thank staff who took on the key worker role for the time and effort they put into the project. We appreciate that for many this was in addition to an already busy workload.

We are grateful to families who were involved in this pilot project, both testing out the key worker service and participating in the project evaluation. We hope that the experience has been worthwhile for all concerned.

During this project we have developed a number of new skills and taken an innovative approach to our work. This was made possible by the advice and encouragement we received from Tricia Norris, our consultant in group work facilitation, and we would like to thank her for her invaluable assistance.

Among the staff at the Social Policy Research Unit, we are grateful to Janet Heaton, Jane Lightfoot, and Rob McMurray for carrying out interviews with families. Finally, we wish to thank Teresa Frank for providing secretarial support to the project, and for remaining calm and cheerful throughout.

1

Introduction

About this report

Key working has the hallmarks of a 'best value' service for families with a disabled child. Parents, researchers, practitioners and policy makers alike have consistently identified the need for key worker services. But how can this be accomplished? The fact that only a minority of families claim to have a key worker reflects the difficulty of providing such a service.

The report is based on the findings of a unique project which sought to open the 'black box' which lies between the notion that offering key workers to families is a 'good thing' and providing such a service. The project involved working with two local authorities - North East Lincolnshire (Site A) and Middlesbrough (Site B) - as they planned, developed and implemented multi-agency pilot key worker services (see Appendix A for further details). Managers and practitioners in these authorities worked in partnership with a research team in order to observe, monitor and evaluate this process, and all those involved in the project, including parents, were interviewed about their experiences of the key worker service.

Overall, the objectives of the project were achieved. Both sites set up pilot key worker services and a considerable amount was learnt about how - and how not - to go about that process. In addition, where individuals had successfully assumed the key worker role, families spoke very highly of the unique support the key worker role offered, and managers and practitioners in both sites were persuaded of its potential benefits.

This report is as much about the failures as the successes observed and recorded during the course of the project, since it is through both that lessons can be learnt. It is concerned with answering broader questions such as 'What is it about key working that families value?' and 'How can multi-agency working be achieved?' But it also seeks to provide readers with the specific, and sometimes practical, details that need to be addressed when planning and developing a key worker service.

There is considerable interest and will to provide families with a disabled child with key workers. From the contacts and conversations we have had over the course of this project it is also very clear that there is a reluctance to 'reinvent the wheel', and a desire to build on and learn from the experiences of those areas where progress has been made on setting up a key worker service. We would not claim that this report holds all the answers, but we do believe it will prove to be a valuable resource to those wishing to move forward the provision of a multi-agency key worker service to families with disabled children in their local area. Certainly the two sites involved in this project will be using it as they move on to 'roll out' their pilot services to a wider range of families with a disabled child in their areas.

Another report has also been written about this project. Entitled *Real change not rhetoric: Putting research into practice in multi-agency services* (Sloper et al, 1999), it is concerned with the process of implementing evidence-based change in social care practice. It describes the innovative approach taken by this project to cross the research-practice divide (something we have called 'researched development work'), and examines the processes involved in developing and implementing change in a multi-agency context.

The concept of key working

Key working is a familiar concept. Since the Court Report in 1976 (DHSS, 1976), it has been repeatedly recommended in legislation and policy guidance documents that key working should form part of the support provided to families with a disabled child. Similarly research consistently reports parents' calls for a 'named person': a single person through which the service maze is accessed and negotiated.

The fact that this same term is defined or applied differently with respect to other groups of service users (for example, adult community care service users, mental health service users) and its very familiarity, makes it worth clarifying what we actually mean by key working for families with a disabled child.

Research into the needs of families with a disabled child and their experiences as service users (for example, Sloper and Turner, 1992; Baldwin and Carlisle, 1994; Beresford, 1994; SSI/Goodinge, 1998), the findings of a quasi-experimental study of key working (Glendinning, 1986), and recent local key working initiatives can be used to identify the scope of the roles and responsibilities of a key worker for a family with a disabled child. The following covers the range of activities that typify the key worker role:

- regular, long-term contact with the family;

- such contact initiated by the key worker, though the family can also make contact at any time;

- provision of information about facilities, opportunities, benefits and entitlements, with respect to both statutory and voluntary agencies;

- identification, through discussions with family members, of the concerns, resources, strengths and needs of the family;

- to advise, support or act on behalf of the family to ensure these needs are met by accessing appropriate services;

- to liaise and improve communication between family members and other professionals/services involved with the family;

- to coordinate the delivery of services and the involvement of other professional workers;

- to participate in decisions made by statutory services concerning service provision to the family, acting as an advocate on the family's behalf.

The distinction between key working and key worker services

Despite its long-standing presence in policy recommendations, parents' demands for such a service, and research evidence to support its effectiveness, *a key worker service* is rarely part of the portfolio of services provided to families with a disabled child (Sloper and Turner, 1992; Beresford, 1995; Chamba et al, 1999). What does seem to happen, however, is that professionals find themselves *key working* on an informal basis with families with whom they are involved

(Cameron and Sturge-Moore, 1990; Baldwin and Carlisle, 1994; Beresford, 1994; While et al, 1996).

This highlights the fact that a *key worker service* is more than just the way an individual professional works with a family. It also includes organisational factors such as the recognition of the role across agencies, and the existence of formal structures to support professionals in this role. Key working can neither be sustained, nor can it be wholly effective, if it is not located within a formal key worker service.

Given these organisational aspects of providing key workers to families with a disabled child, key worker services will differ according to the context, needs, priorities and constraints of the local area in which they are based. As a result there cannot be a specific and rigid formula of what a key worker service should be like and how to set one up. Examples of key worker services currently in operation are described in Appendix C. These show that key working can operate in different contexts and within a range of organisational settings. In all three examples, individuals from a range of professions (health, education and social services) act as key worker for a limited number of families while continuing to work in their other professional role with a much larger caseload. The role of a key worker as a source of support and information, and as a link with statutory services, are common features, as is the notion that contact between families and their key worker should be regular and relatively long term.

Key worker services and multi-agency working

The need to develop and promote working across agencies is a key policy objective as we enter the new millennium. In 1986, Glendinning described key working as 'single door' to all services, across all agencies. Today the notion of key working has once again been implicated as a means of furthering joint working across agencies. A recent government discussion paper (DoH, 1999), argues that a key worker system not only has a role in terms of supporting families but can also promote inter-agency working and collaboration.

Gaining insight, learning lessons - the role of evaluation

A central task of this project was to evaluate the pilot key worker services set up in the two sites participating in the project. In many instances evaluation is seen simply as measuring the effects of an intervention, the key question being did it, or did it not, work? However, such an approach usually generates more questions than answers. In particular, it cannot answer the question *why* something did or did not work.

Pawson and Tilley (1997), among others, advocate an approach to evaluation in which the evaluation of the *process* of implementing or managing an intervention is as important as evaluating the *outcome* of the intervention. This approach is known as *realistic evaluation*. Pawson and Tilley argue: "Programs are *not* things that may (or may not) 'work'; rather they contain certain ideas which work for certain subjects, in certain situations" (1997, p 215).

There are three themes to realistic evaluation. First, realistic evaluation increases the "specificity of our understanding of the mechanisms through which a program accomplishes change" (Pawson and Tilley, 1997, p 114). Second, it enables researchers to examine and identify aspects of the context in which a change or intervention takes place which either support or hinder that change. Third, it increases our ability to predict, based on our understanding of the mechanism and context, the potential outcomes of an intervention or change.

Adopting a realistic approach to evaluation therefore requires seeking the accounts and experiences of all those involved. This includes the *recipients* of the intervention (in our case, the parents); those responsible for carrying out or administering the intervention (the key workers); and those involved in *managing* the development and implementation of the intervention (for instance, service managers). It is also necessary to gather information about the organisational context in which the intervention is taking place.

Such an approach to evaluation, which explored process as well as outcomes, and sought to obtain the views of all involved, was clearly necessary for this project for a number of reasons. First, the intervention (or change) being implemented was taking place in a complex context, and a context known to be fraught with difficulties, namely multi-agency working. Factors within that context may affect the outcomes of the pilot intervention. Furthermore, this context will differ across different sites (that is, local authorities). Second, implementing a key worker service required changing professionals' ways of working - their behaviours and their attitudes. The way that change was managed (that is, the process) would affect the degree to which the new role was accepted and assimilated (Smale, 1996). In addition, the sites differed in the way they managed the development and implementation of the pilot key worker service. Third, the population subject to the intervention (families with a disabled child) is an heterogeneous group. An important feature of key working is that it is individualistic - responding to the specific needs and requests of a family. Any evaluation needs to be able to 'accommodate' this approach.

Finally, and perhaps most important, this project was about *learning*. Learning about setting up and running a key worker service. Learning about problems and solutions throughout the whole process of introducing, supporting and maintaining change. That learning needed to be based on the knowledge gained from asking all parties involved: Did key working achieve its desired outcomes? If so, why? Or, if it did not work, why not? For whom did it work? And in what circumstances did it work? If an evaluation cannot offer answers to these questions its use is extremely limited. For "the strength of evaluation research depends on the perspicacity of its view of explanation" (Pawson and Tilley, 1997, p 219).

The structure of the report

In **Chapter 2** we provide contextual information. This includes the organisational, service and socioeconomic features of the sites involved in the project and the models of key working developed and on which the pilot services were based. We then move on to report the project findings. **Chapter 3** describes the key worker service from the parents' perspective. **Chapter 4** focuses on the experiences of those staff who took on the key worker role. The managers' experiences of managing and implementing the pilot key worker services are reported in **Chapter 5**. In **Chapter 6**, we draw together the evidence. We present a model of key working and summarise the lessons learnt from this project about developing and setting up a key worker service for disabled children and their families. Finally, we offer the guidelines for implementing a key worker service drawn up by the two sites taking part in the project.

2
Contexts and foundations

This chapter provides contextual information, specifically relevant demographic and organisational features, about the two sites involved in this project. It also details the models of key working which the two sites developed for their pilot services and how they approached the implementation of these models. In the previous chapter, we argued the importance of taking into account the context when evaluating and understanding the outcome of an intervention or change. Such information is also important for the reader interested in applying the lessons learnt in the course of this project to their own 'site'.

The demographic and organisational context

We were keen that this project involved two sites with differing demographic and organisational profiles and this was achieved to some degree. Site A was a mixed urban/rural site with pockets of deprivation, while Site B was essentially urban and quite deprived. Although both were unitary authorities, they varied quite considerably in the extent of joint working in place at the beginning of the project in terms of services for disabled children and their families. In Site A, a multi-disciplinary service planning group was meeting regularly in order to develop services provided to families with a disabled child. In contrast, in Site B, while there was a willingness at an individual level to engage in inter-agency working, no joint working or funding structures existed. Further information about the two sites is given in Appendix D.

Models of a pilot key worker service developed by the two sites

An early task for the two sites was to develop a model of the key worker service they wanted to pilot during the course of the project. These models are reproduced in Box 1 (Site A) and Box 2 (Site B). The key worker job descriptions also drawn up by the sites may be found in Appendix E.

Similarities between the two models were that both sites chose to pilot the service with families caring for a child with complex needs, the key workers would be drawn from all three main statutory agencies, and key workers would act as a single point of contact. Both models acknowledged the need for key workers to engage in multi-agency working.

While both models adhere to the basic tenets of key working described in the previous chapter, the functions and ethos of the two pilot key worker services differ somewhat. Site A's model highlighted the importance of empowerment, partnership and an holistic approach. In contrast, Site B emphasised coordination and assessment as the main functions of their pilot service. Another difference between the two sites' models was that one site chose to recruit key workers by a system of volunteering, while the other site identified and approached professionals who were thought to be suitable for the key worker role. The organisational issues identified by the two sites had a differing focus, with only one stating the need for multi-agency commitment. In terms of the aims of the project, one site appeared to be taking a more overt learning approach to the project. We shall return to these similarities and differences in later chapters when we report the services that were put in place.

Implementation of the models

The two sites differed in the size of their pilot service. Site A's steering group was very clear that they wanted to set up a small-scale pilot service through which they could observe and test out the key worker model they had developed. In contrast, the size of the service developed in Site B was decided by the number of professionals volunteering to become pilot key workers.

Box 1: Site A - model of pilot key worker service

Aims of the service
- Provide a key worker service for a small sample of families who are struggling with the complexities of their situation.
- To test out the concept of the key worker model for families of disabled children in this local authority.

Functions of service
- To work in partnership with families to achieve an effective package of services which meets their assessed needs without duplication.
- To empower families to manage their own circumstances as independently as they choose.
- To be a single point of contact for families and agencies as required.

Service provided to...
- Families caring for a child(ren) with a disability who have complex support needs.

Ethos
- Holistic approach to families of child(ren) with a disability.

Professional providing the service
- Representatives from health, education, social services and the voluntary sector.

Training
- Initial induction training.
- Ongoing support will be provided.

Organisational issues
- Commitment from all agencies.
- Set standards for monitoring (with the research team).
- Identifying the key workers.
- Set realistic time-scales.

Box 2: Site B - model of pilot key worker service

Aims of the service

- To provide an identified person who will coordinate and/or facilitate the health and social care, and education for each child with a disability within the pilot group.

Functions of service

- To coordinate and/or facilitate assessment processes and review processes.
- To coordinate the production of a 'plan' which specifies how assessed social, health and education needs will be met.
- To act as a named contact for parents/children and families seeking advice, information, guidance, support, assistance.
- To facilitate communication between agencies and parents and children and families.

Service provided to...

- Families involved with the pre-school assessment unit or using residential short-term care services.
- Child must have a disability.
- Must be receiving services of two or more agencies for at least 12 months.
- Must be willing to take part in pilot project (written consent required).

Ethos

- Enabling families to manage.

Professional providing the service

- Any staff working in the pre-school assessment unit (teachers/nursery nurses).
- Community nurses for children with learning disabilities.
- Social workers - social services department education (specialist social workers).

> ### *Training*
> - Invite people identified as potential key workers to a meeting.
> - Explain aims of the scheme and ask for a minimum of five volunteers.
> - Steering group to arrange training event.
> - Cascade information to other colleagues involved.
>
> ### *Organisational issues*
> - Establish a steering group - representatives from each agency/pilot centres - involve someone from quality assurance for monitoring.
> - Take a paper to joint strategy group for joint funding proposals for a coordinator post to oversee the project.

The key workers

In both sites, the pilot service entailed various professionals taking on the key worker role with one family (or sometimes two families), as opposed to creating designated key worker posts. In some cases, the professional was already working with that family in a different capacity, in others contact was only through the key worker service.

In Site A, members of the steering group identified and approached eight professionals on an individual basis about taking on the role. Site B, in contrast, wrote to staff working in a number of services for children with complex disabilities about the project, and waited to see how many professionals volunteered to become involved. Staff who expressed an interest in becoming a key worker were invited to a one-day meeting to find out more about the project. Here, 19 professionals signed up to becoming a key worker.

'Pilot' key workers included professionals from the main statutory agencies and, in one site, a voluntary agency (see Table 2). In Site A, there was equal representation of health, education and social services. In Site B, the majority of key workers were from social services. In addition, both within and across the agencies, there was a range in terms of the type of professional role represented including: teachers, education welfare officers, residential social workers, social workers, and hospital and community-based nurses.

Table 1: Training and supervision provided to key workers	
Site A	**Site B**
One-day *training* event	One day *information* event
A project coordinator provided:	Steering group provided:
• Regular individual supervision attendance voluntary	• Support group meetings,
• Regular group support meetings	• The offer of a mentor
	• 'Model' case file
	• One supervision session towards end of project

The families

The approach to the recruitment of families paralleled the recruitment of key workers. In Site A, the key workers *selected* a family they would like to work with and asked them to take part in the project. In Site B, families accessing services for children with complex disabilities were asked if they wanted to *volunteer* to take part in the project. Those interested in participating were invited to a meeting with staff and the research team. At these meetings, the key worker service was explained to parents and they had an opportunity to ask questions about the project.

For the purposes of the pilot project, the steering groups in both sites chose to involve families who were already service users. There were a number of reasons for this decision. First, the steering groups wanted to ensure staff acting as key workers were not overburdened; this was more likely to happen if they worked with a family where no services were in place. Second, identifying families to recruit for the pilot would be relatively simple. Third, there were ethical considerations: the steering groups felt it would be inappropriate to test out a new service on families whose child had been newly diagnosed since this was a time when families were likely to be at their most vulnerable.

Management of the pilot service

In Site B, the steering group met monthly over the course of the project and were responsible for the on-going 'day-to-day' management of the

---

Table 2: Professionals key working at the outset and at follow-up

	Site A	Site B
Total number recruited	8 staff: 3 social workers 1 nurse 1 special needs health visitor 1 teacher 1 education welfare officer 1 voluntary sector worker	19 staff: 9 residential social workers 6 field social workers 3 community nurses 1 home manager
Number in contact with families at follow-up interview	8 staff: As above	9 staff: 5 residential social workers 2 field social workers 2 community nurses

pilot. In Site A, the manager of the local multi-disciplinary resource centre for families with a disabled child took on the role of key worker coordinator for the duration of the pilot. A sub-group of the project's steering group, consisting of the managers from health, education and social services, met regularly with the coordinator in order to receive feedback on the progress of the pilot.

Training and supervision

The training and supervision offered to the key workers differed between the two sites (see Table 1).

In Site A, key workers attended a one-day *training* event in which they discussed the role of the key workers, and were introduced to professionals from a range of agencies who they might wish to contact in their role as key worker (for example, leisure, housing, welfare rights). Key workers were also provided with a file containing a wide range of written information about local services and disability benefits. Following the training day, the project coordinator took responsibility for overseeing the key workers, reporting back on their progress to the steering group on a regular basis. The coordinator also provided regular individual supervision sessions and group meetings for key workers.

In Site B, there was an initial one-day *information* event to recruit professionals to the project. At this event, the key worker role was outlined and discussed, and presentations were given on the roles of the different agencies: health, education and social services. In terms of supervision, key workers were invited to attend support group meetings. However, attendance was voluntary and reported to be low. Those who did not attend explained that other work commitments had taken priority. All key workers were given background details on members of the steering group and told they could approach them to be a mentor. This offer was not taken up by any of the key workers. A few months after key workers were allocated to families, staff were given a model case file, outlining the records they should make after each contact with the family. A single supervision session with a member of the steering group was organised for each key worker approximately six months after they were allocated a family.

The status of the pilot services at follow-up

Some 12 months after the start of the project, all eight key workers in Site A reported they were still in contact with families. In Site B, only nine of the original 19 members of staff identified themselves as key workers at the follow-up interview (see Table 2). The reasons for this drop-out rate in Site B are reported in Chapter 4. However, it is important to note at this stage that in all instances professionals left at the beginning of the project rather than after prolonged contact with a family.

3

Key working: parents' reports

In this and the following two chapters, we report the results of this project. We have chosen to organise our findings around the accounts of the three main stakeholders involved: the parents; the professionals who assumed the key worker role; and the managers who developed and implemented the pilot service.

In this chapter, drawing primarily on parents' accounts, we focus on key working in operation. What is happening when a key worker is key working, and how are families experiencing it? In Chapter 4, we report on the experiences of those professionals who took on the key worker role. Finally, Chapter 5 recounts the managers' experiences of implementing the service. These three chapters are very much about reporting results: we reserve our interpretation of our findings to Chapter 6. There we will seek to answer the questions 'Did it work?'; 'Who did it work for?' and 'In what circumstances?'

The parents

Given that we wanted to research the process and outcome of the pilot services, we were keen to involve as many families as possible in the evaluation. However, both sites felt (and we agreed) that it would be unethical to refuse a family a key worker because they were not willing to take part in the evaluation (or research) side of the project. Principally this involvement meant being willing to be interviewed at the end of the pilot period. Six out of the eight families from Site A and 18 out of 19 families from Site B agreed to be involved in the evaluation.

When it came to making contact at the end of the pilot phase, the situation with these 24 families can be seen in Table 3.

The families who had withdrawn from the project did so because they had misunderstood the purpose or role of key workers, or because a change in circumstances made them ineligible for the service. We were unable to contact or interview five families for various reasons

Table 3: The situation of families at the end of the pilot phase

	Site A	Site B
Family assigned key worker and had contact	4	8
Family assigned key worker but no contact	-	1
Family not aware assigned key worker	1	1
Family withdrew from project	-	4
Unable to contact/interview family	1	4
Total	**6**	**18**

including the child being critically ill and/or hospitalisations. A couple of parents did not respond to our letters or telephone calls inviting them to take part in an interview.

The remaining 15 families had been assigned a key worker. Two were unaware that they had been assigned someone to be their key worker. In both instances, the family 'knew' their key worker in another role and spoke of the value of their input. Twelve families were aware they had been assigned a key worker and had been in contact with that individual over the course of the pilot phase. It is data collected from interviews with these 15 families (five in Site A and 10 in Site B) that we report in the remainder of this chapter.

Were the professionals 'key working'?

One of the first questions we had when we examined the parents' accounts was: Were the professionals who had been assigned to be their key worker actually key working? Parents made a judgement as to whether they had received a key worker service based on the information they had received about key working during the course of the project. In particular, parents seemed to focus on two aspects: whether or not the professional was pro-active in making contact with the parents, and whether or not an holistic family-centred approach had been adopted.

Table 4 shows that seven families reported that they had received a key worker service. Two of these parents were unaware of the key worker

Table 4: Extent of key working across families in contact with their key worker at the end of the project

	Site A	Site B
Key worker assigned to family and family report receiving a key worker service	3	2
Parents unaware assigned a key worker but describe receiving a key worker type service from the professional identified by project as their key worker	1	1
Key worker assigned but family report they did not receive a key worker service	1	6

project and denied having a key worker. However, both were in regular contact with the professional assigned by the project to be their key worker and were clearly receiving a key worker service from that professional. (Our interviews with these two professionals revealed a reluctance to introduce the term 'key worker' to families.) A further seven families had had some contact with their key worker but had not, according to them, received a key worker service. From now on in the text we shall refer to this group as 'unsuccessful' key workers.

Parents' perceptions of their experiences are supported by the professionals' responses to the key worker activities questionnaire. Figure 1 demonstrates the differences in the mean scores for a number of key worker activities between key workers and 'unsuccessful' key workers. (It would not be appropriate here to conduct any statistical analysis of these data due to small sample size.)

What the key workers were doing

The specific activities undertaken by key workers were identified from the parents' and their key workers' accounts. The accounts of the parents and key workers were consistent and are summarised in Box 3. The activities described in Box 3 clearly show key working taking place in two 'arenas' - the family context and the organisational context. Described at the top is the supportive and empowering work which goes on within (and for) the *family context*. The context of key working

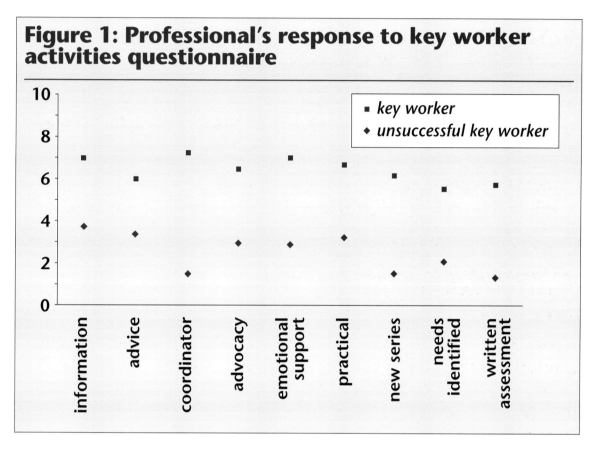

Figure 1: Professional's response to key worker activities questionnaire

activity shifts as we read down the box. In terms of identifying and addressing needs, the key worker is, in a sense, simultaneously working in both family and organisational contexts. Finally, towards the bottom of the box are those activities which happen within an *organisational context*. Here key workers act as the 'bridge' between other professionals/ services and the family, playing a role in service coordination and being a source of information for other professionals working with the family. Figure 2 offers a simple pictorial representation of the ways in which the two key working contexts are either overlapping or are distinct, depending on the specific key working activity.

What is important to stress here is that the organisational context in which key workers were working was not a single-agency context. Key workers reported working in a *multi-agency context*, involving liaison with other professionals both within their own agency and in other agencies. Having named contacts and advice on how to best approach different agencies made multi-agency working easier for key workers in Site A.

Box 3: Activities undertaken by key workers

Emotional support

- Listening.
- Offering an objective/rational insight into a problem.
- Affirming parents' ways of managing or dealing with their situation.

Information and advice to the family

- Obtaining information - regarding services, child's condition, etc.
- Providing advice on managing specific problems faced by the family.

Identifying and addressing needs

- Identifying needs of all family members (but not formal needs assessment).
- Accessing or assisting with applications for new services or other forms of support across the statutory and voluntary sectors.
- Assisting and empowering families to access services themselves.
- Facilitating parents to explore solutions to particular difficulties/needs which cannot be met by forms of statutory support.

Advocacy

- Acting as an advocate for the family in a wide range of meetings with professionals - either speaking on their behalf and/or supporting parents to act as their own advocates.
- Assisting family in their dealings with agencies.

Coordination

- Involvement in coordinating new or existing care packages.
- Providing other professionals with information about the family.
- Liaising/acting as a link between the family and other professionals.

Differences in key working between families

So far we have provided an overall picture of the range of activities key workers undertook. There were, however, considerable differences between families in terms of the nature of input and support provided by the key worker. Analysis of families' responses to the key worker activities questionnaire administered at the end of the pilot illustrates

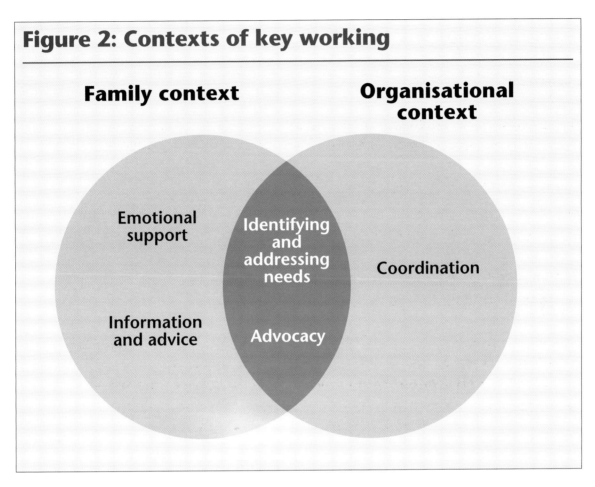

Figure 2: Contexts of key working

Family context

Organisational context

Emotional support

Identifying and addressing needs

Coordination

Information and advice

Advocacy

this (see Figure 3). In this figure, the mean score is indicated by the diamond shape. The lines extending through the diamond indicate the minimum and maximum scores for each dimension.

Overall, this figure shows a high level of involvement with most key working activities, with parents reporting key workers being least involved in providing written assessments. In addition, parents report a greater level of involvement with tasks or support which take place in the family context, as opposed to activities which are undertaken in the organisational context, such as accessing new services and service coordination. This will, in part, be due to families' greater awareness of activities stemming from direct contact with their key worker, as opposed to the tasks undertaken on their behalf but not in their presence.

A very striking message from these data is the enormous variation between parents' reports within each of the defined key worker

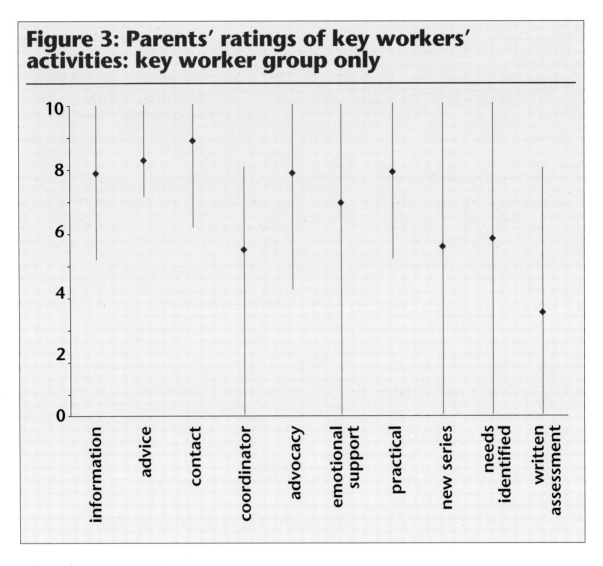

Figure 3: Parents' ratings of key workers' activities: key worker group only

activities. Analysis of the interviews with parents suggests a number of reasons for this. First, it reflects the considerable individual differences in families' needs and strengths, and hence the types of support they wanted from their key worker. This, we would argue, highlights the need for key working to adopt a flexible, individualistic approach. Second, one or two parents were very conscious of the organisational constraints and lack of resources and/or services within which their key worker was having to operate. We return to both these points later in the chapter.

Having a key worker: its unique value

Earlier, we reported that seven families worked with, and were supported by, professionals who had truly assumed the key worker role.

All these parents spoke highly of the work and support their key worker had provided to their families. Furthermore, families in the 'unsuccessful' key worker group, who through their involvement with the project had learned about the notion of key working, felt that key workers should be an *integral* part of services provided to families with a disabled child.

The reasons behind this very positive experience (or perception) of key working can be found in the parents' accounts - both those in the key worker and 'unsuccessful' key worker groups. Some very consistent themes or issues emerged which we have found helpful to think about as the six *elements of key working*. These are:

- pro-active, regular contact;

- a supportive, open relationship;

- a family-centred approach;

- working across agencies;

- working with families' strengths and ways of coping;

- working for the family as opposed to working for an agency.

This conceptualisation of key working is not describing, at the micro level, particular tasks and activities a key worker might undertake for a family. Rather it is concerned with the generic role of key working, offering a broader context in which to understand the specific, individualistic key working which may be done in partnership with a particular family, as well as highlighting the differences that exist between this role and other professional roles.

The elements of key working

Pro-active, regular contact

Having regular contact initiated by the key worker was an extremely positive experience for parents. As we noted earlier, the presence or absence of pro-active contact by the professional assigned to the family was the main dimension along which parents appeared to judge whether or not they had received a key worker service. The following excerpts are taken from interviews with two parents in the 'unsuccessful' key worker group. This first statement highlights the difficulty some parents have in asking for help until they are 'in crisis':

> "When somebody gives you a card and says 'Ring me if you need me' it doesn't help. Because if they are anything like me they'll struggle on without asking for help, because people do."

> "The way it worked was that we would contact her if we needed anything. I would have preferred someone who would have contacted us and said 'Hey, what about this?' … someone a bit more pro-active."

The frequency of this pro-active contact - and the form it took - varied between families and was something that needed to be negotiated between the key worker and family.

A supportive, open relationship

Parents in the key worker group described their relationship with their key worker as being different from their relationship with other professionals. The word friend or friendship was often used by parents to describe the relationship between themselves and their key worker. This was based on a belief that the key worker knew more about the parents or family than might have been divulged to other professionals, and that there was a sense of trust that allowed parents to be honest or open with their key worker:

> "Yes, it's as though I was talking to a neighbour. A very close neighbour, well - a friend. Someone that I can say to 'bloody [name of child] has done this and that...'. I can really moan to her."

It was clear to parents that such a relationship takes time to develop. A parent in the 'unsuccessful' key worker group described how she wished her 'key worker' had taken time to get to know her and her family, to know the parent 'as a person and not just a number'. This parent observed it would take time and regular contact before she would feel able to approach her 'key worker'.

> "... it's important that there is someone there that you can relate to and have a trust with ... trust is very important. There isn't a relationship [with my 'key worker']. There's nothing there. If she rings you feel suspicious. You wonder why she's ringing."

Parents felt that the domiciliary nature of the service promoted or supported greater equality in the key worker-family relationship.

> "I would want my key worker to phone me more to see if things are okay rather than wait for us to go to [the key worker's place of work]. To take it out of the workplace and become more of a friend of the family."

A family-centred as opposed to a child-centred approach

The third feature which contributes to the distinctive nature of key working was the family-centred approach adopted by professionals undertaking a key working role. Acknowledging and seeking to address the needs of all family members was seen as very different to parents' other experiences of statutory support.

> "I think the difference with [my key worker] is that she's the type of person who wants us to have what we should have. [My key worker] looks at it differently to other professionals. She thinks about the need to improve my life and my other child's life as well as my disabled child's life. She looks at everything in terms of trying to find things that would make our lives easier."

This following account of an essentially child-centred approach offers an important contrast in terms of the parents' experiences. This parent was assigned a 'key worker' who already worked with the family in another role:

> "She [key worker] doesn't know me. She knows my child because [child] goes in for [service]. But she doesn't know what my specific needs are, or where my specific areas of help are needed with [all] my children or anything like that."

Finally, parents believed that the fact that their key worker visited them at home promoted a family-centred approach. It meant the key worker was more likely to see other members of the family, hence encouraging a more holistic, family-centred approach. In addition, the physical and social context in which the family was living was very apparent.

Working across agencies

Adopting a family-centred approach necessarily drives key working into working across agencies, and being able to contact one person about *any* issue was highly valued by parents. This engendered a sense among parents of being supported. It also relieved them of the not inconsiderable problem of discovering who they needed to contact or where they needed to go about a specific problem.

> "What I like is that I can ring her and it doesn't matter what it is. She's there for you. She's very supportive."

> "I think top of the list is to know that there's somebody there ... the reassurance that you know someone's there willing to listen to you. And the thought that if you can't get something done she'll know somebody that can - she'll know some other way around it, who to write to, who to phone."

We must not underestimate the importance parents place on knowing there is one person they can turn to:

> "I'm a very independent person but you still need the thought that you've got someone you can turn to."

Thus from the families' perspective, an important aspect of key working is to facilitate service coordination and inter-agency working. This is something that families find extremely difficult to do by themselves, as this parent's account shows:

> "I was going from one person to another, tearing myself in shreds and getting nowhere. I wanted someone to be at the front for me. I was fed up with one lot of professionals telling me my child was 'social' and the other lot saying she was 'health', and meanwhile I'm in the middle getting nothing. So instead of me going to these horrendous meetings and being torn apart by people, I wanted someone else to go and do the nasty bits and come back and give me the good news.

Which is what [my key worker] does! She's been excellent. I can't praise her enough. I've been able to take a back seat. I've been relieved of the stress, someone else has been there to take it for me."

It is, however, not only a question of working across agencies in terms of coordinating services already in place. There is a role for key workers at an earlier stage in terms of knowing what different agencies, or services within agencies, might be able to offer a family, knowing how to go about accessing them, and then giving that information to parents for them to act on, or to act on their behalf.

This is the response one parent gave when asked why she had decided to have a key worker:

"I thought it would be a good idea. Dealing with all the services - health, social security, social services and education - it can be a nightmare getting the right information. So having someone to help sort it out or give us new information we hadn't come across, that would be useful."

Similarly, it might not be that the key worker assumes a *lead* role in service coordination. As we discussed earlier, the key workers in this study were not reported to be heavily involved in the more organisational aspects of key working. Thus for some families it was simply a case of their key worker knowing who to get in touch with, 'getting the ball rolling' rather than actually managing or directing coordination. Obviously this depended on the inter-agency context in which the key workers were working.

Working with families' strengths and ways of coping

In an earlier section, we highlighted the fact that the tasks or roles undertaken by key workers varied quite considerably between families. One of the reasons underlying this was that families have different needs and problems. In addition, families also differ in the skills, experience and expertise they bring to their situation. With respect to the issue of key working, the most notable area of difference between parents was the degree to which they wanted to advocate for themselves, and the skills and networks they had developed with respect to this prior to being assigned a key worker. Another, somewhat related, area of difference concerned the frequency at which parents wanted regular, pro-active contact from their key worker.

> "I think our key worker understands that we like to do things off our own back, that we're not on the 'phone everyday. We discussed this right at the start."

Identifying parents' strengths and preferred ways of coping and then negotiating with them as to the support and input needed from the key worker is an important part of developing an effective partnership between parents and key workers.

Working for the family and not an agency

Finally, and perhaps the culmination of the previous elements, is that parents who had been key worked did not regard their key worker as operating within a certain professional role or within a particular agency. This was extremely important in terms of the key worker's ability to act as an advocate for the family:

> "That someone is there for me, for my interests, not acting for social services or whatever. As a parent that's really good."

At the same time, the importance of having a professional (someone, sadly, with greater status than parents within the context of statutory agencies) acting as their advocate was stressed by parents.

> "Because she's a professional she can take things to a higher level. She got it sorted out. She knew who to 'phone and what to say. Whereas, as a parent, I would have just got on the phone and shouted at somebody. As a professional you can always stand back, you're not so much in the heat of it. Everything runs so smoothly now compared to a year or even six months ago."

Some parents wanted to be their own advocates. Having a key worker supporting them 'behind the scenes', ready to step in if necessary, was reassuring and empowering.

> "I'm quite happy to do things on my own, but I've got to know that [my key worker] is there in the background if I become unstuck ...

[it's having] a professional in the background. Somebody who other people, other professionals, will take notice of."

Parents' suggestions and recommendations

In this final section we will report parents' ideas and suggestions about key working - both in terms of who should be a key worker and who most needs a key worker, and also around organisational issues which need to be addressed in order to support key working. We begin with the latter.

The organisational context and supporting key working: parents' views

We analysed parents' views and recommendations working from the premise that a suitable, well-trained key worker has been assigned to a family. Our question was, what were parents' views about how the organisations or agencies involved can ensure effective key working takes place? Three themes emerged:

- when acting as advocates, key workers need to be 'independent' of statutory agencies;

- ensuring parents understand what key working is;

- ensuring a 'cover' key worker is available.

The need to be 'independent' of statutory agencies when advocating for a family

One or two families had been in situations when, as acting as their advocate, their key worker had faced conflict between their role as key worker and their other role. This proved to be a difficult experience, both for the key worker and the parents. For the parents, it highlighted the need to protects and respect professionals 'independence', both from their statutory responsibilities and their responsibilities to their employer, when advocating for a family. The pen portrait illustrates this point.

Pen portrait: managing a conflict of interests

Mrs Campbell's key worker was also her social worker. Mrs Campbell had been 'battling' for a year and a half to improve the heating in her home, and this had culminated in Mrs Campbell being asked to attend a tribunal (against social services). The key worker was told by her manager that she could not come to the tribunal to support Mrs Campbell since it would represent a social worker going against social services. Having talked it over with her key worker, Mrs Campbell rang her key worker's manager (in social services) stating that her key worker would be attending the tribunal as her key worker and not as her social worker, "I said I had the right to have someone with me, so they couldn't refuse then". At the tribunal Mrs Campbell noted that her key worker had to be very careful not to cross over from the key worker role to the social worker role. Mrs Campbell recalled that "it was a very emotional time".

Ensuring parents understand what key working is

A reason for a couple of the key worker-parent relationships breaking down in this pilot study was because parents had been misinformed, or misunderstood what the role of their key worker would be, and the type of help and support they could and could not offer. This led to unnecessary confusion, disappointment and disillusionment.

This highlights the more general point that key working might not only be a new way of working for professionals, it also has the potential to positively transform parents' expectations of professional or statutory support. As with any change or anything new, individuals need information, in order both to decide whether or not they need that sort of help, and so that such help can be used most effectively.

Ensuring a 'cover' key worker is available

One parent specifically mentioned the need to provide cover or back-up when the key worker is not available (for example, on holiday, sick or maternity leave). This parent encountered a particularly difficult and unpleasant situation while her key worker was on holiday, and found that there was nobody else who could help her. Ideally, parents should have met the 'cover key worker'.

"A back-up person would be good. It would be good if you had met such a person face-to-face just once, so you knew who they were."

About key working: parents' recommendations

Parents had a number of ideas and suggestions about who should be a key worker and who most needs a key worker.

Who should be a key worker?

The qualities necessary in a good key worker and key workers' training or information needs were discussed by parents.

In terms of ideal key worker qualities, certain personality traits or ways of interacting were mentioned by parents. These included: patient, understanding, empathetic, reliable, approachable and non-judgemental. In addition to describing these particular characteristics, parents drew attention to the importance of the key worker and the family 'getting on' in order that the sort of relationship we have described above can be fostered. One parent commented that "... people should be matched up well".

Specific skills or information needs included: being able to diffuse emotional situations; having a detailed knowledge of the local 'system' - the roles and responsibilities of different agencies, knowing how to work across agencies, and about available services; and more general knowledge of the rights and entitlements of disabled children and their families. In addition, parents felt that a grounding in what is known about the needs of families with a disabled child, as well as an understanding of disabilities and impairments, were both important.

"My key worker has specialist knowledge about social services, she doesn't necessarily have any knowledge about health or education that parents also need. So a key worker would ideally have a broader background and experience, or get that through training."

Who should get a key worker?

Parents identified both *types of family* and *stages in the family life cycle* when having a key worker would be especially pertinent.

Single parents, or those living in unsupportive relationships, were seen by some (not only the single parents) as particularly needing a 'professional' partner with whom to work through and work out solutions to their situation.

Another way of 'prioritising' who should have a key worker centred on the stage a family was at. Two periods - diagnosis and transition to adult services - were reported by parents as being times when having a key worker could make a tremendous difference to families.

Key findings

- In terms of parents' reports, at the time of follow-up, professionals who had taken on the role of key worker for this project could be classified as key workers or 'unsuccessful' key workers. The extent of regular pro-active contact and a family-centred (as opposed to child-centred) approach were the two main factors informing parents' judgements about the service they had received.

- Families in the key worker group described the service they received very positively and perceived it to be different to other forms of support they had experienced.

- Overall, the aspects of the key working which appeared to be important to families' positive reports of the service they received were as follows:

  - pro-active regular support;
  - a supportive, open relationship;
  - a family-centred approach;
  - working across agencies;
  - working with families' strengths and ways of coping;
  - working for the family as opposed to working for an agency.

- However, there were differences between families on the emphasis needed (or given) to each of these elements. This was both a reflection of a particular family's strengths and needs as well as the organisational context in which the key working was taking place.

- Parents highlighted the need for key workers to be able to be independent of their employer or statutory agencies when acting as an advocate.

- There was consensus among parents that the period immediately after diagnosis was the stage at which they would have most valued having a key worker. Single parents were also identified as a group who might particularly need the support that can be offered through a key worker service.

4

The experience of being a key worker

In this chapter we describe the experience of the staff who were recruited into the project as key workers (see Table 2). We begin by outlining their views on the project at the outset. We then track the experiences of those who were recruited into the project but who were not key working at the time of the follow-up interview. The rest of the chapter focuses on the experiences of those who were key working, including:

- perceptions of the key working role;

- the advantages of taking on the role;

- the difficulties encountered;

- views on the service implementation;

- recommendations on the future of the service in their area.

Views at the outset

Attitudes towards participation in the project

From the start of the project, the attitudes of staff towards participation in the project were very different in the two sites. This seemed to stem from the recruitment process. In Site A, staff were selected by the steering group and asked to take part in the project. They included staff from health, education, social services, and the voluntary sector (see Table 2). When asked why they were participating in the project, they said they felt obliged to since they had been asked to by their line manager. Most could see no difference between the key worker role and what they did in their everyday work with families, apart from the possibility that the frequency of their contacts with the family and other agencies might increase.

In Site B, the steering group *invited* all members of staff from a number of services within health, education and social services to take part in the project. They said they 'sold' the project to staff as an opportunity to gain experience and training not otherwise available. The staff who volunteered were predominantly from social services. Unlike in Site A, many were working in a residential setting. The remaining key workers were drawn from health services. None were recruited from education. Those who agreed to participate did so because they liked the key worker concept, and saw it as a challenge and an opportunity to develop new skills. Only one person mentioned feeling "pushed into taking part". Very few staff had difficulty distinguishing between their everyday work and the key worker role.

Concerns

Despite their differences in attitude towards participating in the project, staff in both sites had a number of common concerns about taking on the key worker role which, in the event, did not prove to be problematic. These included:

- concerns that the service might disempower parents;

- that families might have high expectations;

- that the key worker could get too emotionally involved with the family;

- that other professionals would think that the key worker was 'taking over'.

Later in the chapter we describe the actual problems key workers faced and their attempts to overcome them.

Failure to establish key working

At the end of Chapter 2, we described the status of the two pilot services when the follow-up evaluation was conducted, some nine to 12 months after they had been set up. In Site A, it appeared that all the key workers were still engaged in this role. However, in Site B half the professionals who had volunteered to take part in the project were not key working at the follow-up interview. There were a variety of reasons why 10 people in Site B were not key working at the follow-up interview. These fell into two main categories: problems in recruitment of families, and key worker difficulties in carrying out the key worker role.

Problems in recruitment of families

One key worker discovered the family she was allocated had a child who had recently been transferred on to adult services, thus making them ineligible for the key worker service. Two families decided for themselves that they did not want a key worker after having an initial meeting to find out about the service. Finally, two families did not respond to key workers' attempts to make contact through telephone calls, letters and home visits.

Difficulties assuming the key worker role

One person reported that she had simply not got around to contacting the family she had been allocated. Two key workers went on long-term leave (sick leave and maternity leave) and did not resume contact with the family on return to work. Replacement cover was not organised for either family. In a further two cases, key workers appear not to have received the necessary training and support to take on the role. In these instances, key workers reported that they had made contact with their family but the relationship had quickly broken down due to a number of difficulties, including:

- problems in communicating with a family for whom English was a second language;

- colleagues failing to pass on messages from the family;

- not feeling equipped to deal with the families' needs, for example, obtaining adaptions and benefits;

- difficulties in finding time for the role;

- tension between the family and the key worker due to the key worker feeling she was being asked to take on tasks she considered inappropriate to the role.

In one case, the difficulties culminated in the family asking to be allocated a different key worker, and the key worker was replaced. In the other case, the key worker referred the family on to social services and ceased contact.

The experience of being a key worker

In this section, we describe the experiences of those staff who identified themselves as key workers at the follow-up interview. Key working is often portrayed in the literature and policy/practice guidance as a very different way of supporting families with a disabled child, compared to more common patterns of crisis intervention and short-term support. It was important for us to find out the views of the professionals who had taken on this role. Furthermore, one of the aims of the project was to investigate the problems and opportunities in implementing key worker services. It was important to explore both what benefits there were for staff in taking on the role and what difficulties they encountered.

Professionals' perceptions of the key working role

Half the key workers in each site had some difficulty in seeing differences between the key worker role and their everyday work. These included key workers from a range of professional backgrounds, including teachers, social workers, residential social workers and community nurses. However, when probed further, most key workers were able to list at least one difference between what they did as key worker and their everyday work. These included:

- more frequent contact with families;

- being pro-active in contacting families;

- families approaching them for assistance;

- liaison with agencies not normally approached;

- helping families with things that affect them within the home;

- taking on an advocacy role;

- being the families' main point of contact;

- being responsive to the families' needs;

- meeting with the family in the home or hospital setting.

Even after extensive probing, there were two people who maintained that what they did as a key worker was no different from their everyday work. In one instance, the key worker had been allocated a family who seemed to have little need for a key worker service, so little support had been provided. In the other case, the key worker was a care manager for children with life-threatening illness and saw the roles as essentially the same.

The advantages of being a key worker

Two types of advantages were reported: improvements to multi-agency working and relationships with parents. Interestingly, only key workers in Site A reported benefits in terms of multi-agency working. These included increased understanding of how professionals in other agencies worked and the problems they encountered; developing closer links with other professionals; and easier access to services.

In terms of relationships with parents, key workers spoke of enjoying the opportunity to work more closely with families than usual; having a better understanding of the difficulties parents encountered; and learning what could be done for a family, given the time to work more intensely.

The difficulties encountered by key workers

At the second interview, some of the concerns raised at the outset of the project remained and other difficulties not anticipated were encountered. These are reported below.

Having time for the role

While having time for the role was the most common concern among key workers at the first interview, in practice, many key workers found that this was not an issue. Families were often not as demanding as staff had expected. Some key workers managed to find allocated time for the role by becoming the family's social worker or by negotiating time for the role when their job was reviewed. However, a few key workers mentioned doing some of their key working tasks outside of work time. One key worker who had a particularly demanding family described the experience as "draining, emotionally, mentally, and physically".

The need for non-contact time

Key workers spoke of the need to leave their usual work place when taking on the key worker role, in order to liaise with other professionals and to make home visits. This was difficult for staff whose usual job involved spending most of their time working directly with children.

Maternity and sick leave

Key workers in both sites were concerned about how the service could provide cover for maternity and long-term sick leave, since no cover had been provided while they were on leave.

Professionals taking on key working as an additional role

Key workers had concerns about taking on a dual role with families; acting as their key worker and continuing to be involved in another professional capacity, for example, as their social worker or education welfare officer. Their prime concern was that this created confusion, since staff and families had difficulty knowing in what capacity the person was working with the family. Staff also reported conflict between their professional statutory responsibilities and the key worker role, where the focus is on supporting the family.

Training and supervision

As outlined in Chapter 2, the training and supervision provided for key workers was different in the two sites. However, staff in both sites mentioned difficulties due to not understanding the key worker role and the type of support they were expected to offer families. Overall, lack of training and supervision was more of an issue for key workers in Site B. The specific comments about training and supervision in each site were as follows:

Site A: Key workers were positive about the training and support they received. Those who attended the training day particularly appreciated being given a list of named contacts in each agency. All key workers were positive about the individual supervision they received from the project coordinator, commenting that it helped to keep them on track as to what they were meant to be doing, and that the supervisor had been helpful in meeting with and writing to the family and other professionals, and in making himself available outside of scheduled supervision sessions.

Key workers particularly valued group meetings, reporting that they had been "like a good inter-agency meeting". The meetings were reported to be supportive through making individuals aware that they were not alone in experiencing difficulties with the role; providing useful ideas on how to solve problems; and giving them access to information they would not normally receive about other agencies and services.

However, key workers did identify some areas where they would have liked more training. Three people said they needed more input on what the key worker role entailed, the situations they would face and how to deal with them. Further training days were also suggested to update people on changes to benefits and to re-motivate key workers.

Site B: There was a clear view in Site B that more training and supervision was needed. Despite the fact that few people had attended support group meetings, they said there was a need for such meetings. However, they specified that key workers should have been allocated time to attend these meetings. They also suggested that these meetings ought to involve more than people just sharing experiences - there should have been someone at the meeting they could go to with queries. Secondly, supervision should have been provided by people experienced in offering this type of support at an early point in the project, and focused on clarifying the key worker role. This early supervision should have been followed up with regular sessions. Finally, key workers felt there should have been more training on what was expected from key workers, particularly for those who entered the project late; how to deal with financial issues, including Disability Living Allowance; how to access occupational therapy and sort out adaptations; and how to set up a joint care plan between social services, health and education.

Key workers' views on the service implementation

During the course of our interviews, key workers were asked about the way in which the service had been implemented in their area and for any suggestions on how the implementation of services might have been approached differently. Interestingly, similar issues arose in both sites: the recruitment of key workers; the allocation of key workers to families; and the relationship between the steering group and key workers.

Recruitment of key workers

Key workers in both sites thought it was important that staff volunteer for the role of key worker.

The allocation of key workers to families

There were mixed views on whether families should have been matched with a member of staff they already knew. Those who had been allocated a family they had never met before said that it took a long time for them to get to know the family and other professionals, and that the family got confused about their role. However, those already involved with the family prior to the project said this led to a feeling that there was little need to contact the family in the role as key worker.

Awareness-raising

In Site A, it was suggested that it might have been helpful if the steering group members had done more work to raise the profile of the project among middle management. This was considered particularly important within social services, so that managers understand what key working involves and do not perceive it as a criticism of existing social work practice.

The relationship between the steering group and key workers

In both sites, key workers felt there could have been more communication between the steering groups and key workers. As it was, key workers felt that decisions were made without prior consultation. In addition, staff in Site A would have liked some feedback from the steering group on the work they were undertaking. In Site B, key workers wanted to be properly informed when support meetings were being held and to be forewarned that they were to receive supervision. On a more positive note, key workers in Site B appreciated the fact that the steering group had given them background information and contact details on all members of the group.

Key workers' views on future involvement in the service

All staff who were recruited into the project were asked if they wanted to make any recommendations about the future of key worker services in their area. In both sites, it was suggested that any future service should be offered to families who were most in need of such support, such as those whose child had recently been diagnosed. In addition, some key workers suggested it would make for an efficient use of resources if key workers were only offered to families who do not have a social worker since the two roles are so similar.

In Site A, key workers were not keen to continue with the role themselves, with only one person mentioning that they would like to see the service maintained as it was. Two people argued that there was little need for a key worker service since the role was similar to what many staff, particularly social workers, undertook as part of their everyday work.

In Site B, despite the difficulties some had experienced, almost all key workers supported the idea of having a key worker service. They acknowledged that there were problems with the current service and recommended that those involved in organising the service try to sort these out and continue:

> "There needs to be a recognition that the project is here and going to work. This has not happened yet. I don't think people are excited about it. There is a bit of doom and gloom about it. That's a pity because there are a lot of positive things about it."

Key findings

- At the outset of the project, staff in Site A felt *obliged* to take part, whereas staff in Site B *volunteered* because they liked the key worker concept and saw it as an opportunity to develop new skills.

- Ten staff in Site B reported that they were not in contact with their allocated family due to problems in the recruitment of families or difficulties in assuming the key worker role.

- The advantages in taking on the key worker role were:

    - improvements in multi-agency working for staff in Site A;
    - improvements in relationship with parents.

- Difficulties encountered by key workers were:

    - not having enough time for the role;
    - the need to spend time outside their usual workplace;
    - the difficulty of finding replacement cover during maternity or sick leave;
    - the confusion created by being involved with a family both as their key worker and in another professional capacity;
    - lack of training and supervision.

- In relation to service implementation, key workers suggested that:

    - staff should volunteer for the role;
    - that the profile of a key worker service needs to be raised among middle management;
    - that there is regular communication between key workers and those steering the service implementation.

- In the future, key workers suggested the service be offered to families at the point of diagnosis.

5

Developing and implementing a key worker service: the managers' perspectives

In this chapter we present the views of the managers who developed and implemented the service in the two case sites. This account is based on interviews with a sub-group of managers from both steering groups which were held towards the end of the project, some two years after the managers first met with the research team and agreed to develop a key worker service in their area. We tried to interview a representative from health, education and social services in each steering group (see Table 5). Unfortunately, it was not possible to interview a manager from education services in Site B.

The findings from each site are presented separately in order to give a clear overview of the implementation process in each area. We open

---

Table 5: Managers interviewed about the development and implementation of the key worker service

Site A

Education	Principal Education Officer - Special Needs
Health trust	General Manager, Family Service
Social services	Assistant Director of Social Services
Joint-funded post	Key Worker Project Coordinator

Site B

Social services	Manager of Children's Services
	Services Manager, Children and Families
	Team Manager, Children's Disability Services
Health authority	Commissioning Manager

with managers' views on the contextual factors which influenced the service implementation. This is followed by an overview of the steering group's role, including any difficulties encountered and suggestions as to how, with hindsight, they might have approached the implementation differently. Finally, we present reflections on the key worker model developed in their area.

Site A

Contextual influences

Generally, the managers felt that the context in which the project had been introduced had been helpful to the project. First, there was a genuine commitment among the steering group members to developing a key worker service. The site was a relatively new unitary authority, with managers who were motivated to develop multi-agency working. Second, there was already some multi-agency working: managers on the steering group were meeting regularly through other multi-agency planning groups and had developed a good working relationship. Third, the organisational structure of the site was said to have helped: the health trust was coterminus with the local authority, which meant less people needed to be involved in decision making. Fourth, shortly after the first workshop, the steering group appointed a project coordinator. This was said to have happened more by luck than design since a new multi-agency disability service was being set up in the area and there was some flexibility about what roles the coordinator of this service took on. It was arranged that the coordinator would provide ongoing training and supervision to key workers and meet with managers on the steering group regularly to update them on key workers' progress. Managers reported that the coordinator was an important link with the key workers, though one person was concerned that they had perhaps relied on this link too much and should have had more meetings with key workers.

The steering group role

The steering group was described as taking a learning approach to implementation, launching the project on a small scale, allowing time to reflect on progress. Managers felt that such an approach was beneficial, suggesting they would not have learnt as much from the project if they had been too preoccupied with directing it. In terms of the steering group input, managers reported that they had:

- steered the project's direction;

- ensured it kept on track;

- ensured continued support at a high level within the organisation;

- given the project status;

- engaged local agencies so as to maintain a multi-agency approach;

- liaised with relevant external agencies, for example, Barnardo's and the research team.

They reported that this had been an exciting process to be involved in.

Difficulties encountered in implementation

Managers reported that it was difficult to find staff to take on the key worker role since it was perceived as arduous. This meant they had to ensure staff were given extra time for the job. It was particularly difficult to find key workers from education services, primarily because these staff spent most of their time working directly with children, leaving little time for key worker responsibilities.

Managers felt they had underestimated the importance of the personal skills of the staff who took on the key worker role, and the time it would take to develop these skills. The fact that staff reported the role as stressful was taken as an indication of the need for more training in negotiation, time-management and assertiveness skills than it had been possible to offer during the course of the project.

Reflections on managing change and implementation

Reflecting on the steering group role, there were a number of things managers felt they should have done differently.

There should have been a bigger launch of the project to professionals
This would have ensured that other professionals were clearer about the purpose of the key worker service.

More regular meetings with key workers to review progress were needed

This would have ensured that specific problems were brought to the steering group's attention early on.

A clearer key worker model and job description

The model needed to be more specific about the boundaries of the key worker role, particularly what tasks key workers should not undertake themselves but could pass on to other professionals, and how regularly they should be in contact with families.

The project coordinator's experience

The coordinator said he had learnt a lot from taking on the role, particularly about the issues faced by families on a daily basis. However, he did have some concerns about the basis on which he was involved in the project. First, he said that ideally he would like to have been involved with the project from the beginning since there were some aspects of the model he did not feel were ideal. Second, he reported that adding the role on to his job had worked for the pilot project in the short term, but a dedicated person would be needed if the service was extended, since key workers required regular training sessions.

The project coordinator viewed senior managers' sustained involvement in the steering group as crucial to the project. He explained that if managers had not attended workshops and meetings it would have seemed they were not interested. However, they had consistently attended such events, making it clear to key workers that the project was important to the authority.

Strengths of the key worker model

The managers in Site A felt there were two main strengths to their model. First, having a project coordinator who took on line manager responsibilities, monitored progress and coordinated the service, was thought to have been vital. It was recommended that any key worker service include such a person, since staff needed to be monitored and given some direction.

Second, the fact that key workers were drawn from health, education, social services and the voluntary sector, meant that a 'reservoir of expertise' was available within the key worker group. At group meetings, key workers could raise the problems they were experiencing and there was always someone within the group who could offer advice.

However, there were two aspects of the model which the steering group felt required further thought and some adjustment.

Should the key worker role be added on to another job?

Managers remained unsure whether key working should be added on to another role, as had been the case for the project. They pointed out that the education sector's (particularly teachers') ability to provide the service was limited due to constraints on staff time. The role was also problematic for social workers, who were reported to be struggling to differentiate between the social work and key worker role. More generally, the key worker role in supporting the family was reported to conflict with the statutory responsibilities held by many professionals.

The time span of the service

One of the aims in this site was that the services offered to families should not be time-limited. Instead, families should have a person they could turn to about their support needs during the course of their child's development. However, in practice it had been difficult for key workers to sustain contact with families when there were long periods when families needed little support. The idea of a life-time service for families was also thought to make key workers feel anxious since it was resource intensive. An alternative suggestion was that the role should be limited to a series of tasks. Once these were completed the key worker could move on to another family.

Site B

Contextual influences

Managers reported that there was a lot of energy and enthusiasm among staff at the start of the project. This was attributed to the site being a new unitary authority keen to develop joint working. This enthusiasm for joint working was fuelled by a push at a national level to be more creative about service organisation. The project also fitted in with the increasing pressure to listen to service users: parents were repeatedly telling professionals that they needed a single point of contact.

However, there were a number of contextual factors which had a negative influence on the implementation. First, managers explained that local services were working in a single agency manner. This made it difficult to implement a multi-agency key worker service, since individual key workers tended to work according to their own agency's agenda. As a result, managers felt they needed to have multi-disciplinary disability teams in place before they could set up a mainstream key worker service. They could then ask staff in these teams to take on the key worker role.

Furthermore, as the project progressed, staff workloads increased because of the number of the government initiatives being taken on and financial constraints within departments. As a result the project became less of a priority, with steering group members focusing on the more fundamental elements of their work.

Finally, four people (one from education, three from social services) were lost from the steering group during the course of the project. One of these people had lead responsibility for the project and was replaced, but the other three members were not, so the group became smaller. Extensive restructuring within education also meant a change of job for the local education authority representative on the group, which resulted in her being less powerful in supporting education's involvement in the latter stages of the implementation of the service. The local education authority's limited involvement in the project was also reported to have contributed to difficulties in recruiting key workers from education services.

The steering group role

The steering group was reported to be the driving force behind the project: defining its parameters as planning, coordinating, monitoring progress, and trouble shooting. Having an action plan and time-scale for events was reported to have helped to keep the steering group focused about the purpose of the project.

Difficulties encountered in implementation

Managers reported that professionals' concerns about the time they would have to spend on the project led to the steering group "nearly begging people to do it". This had been one of the reasons why they had accepted all volunteers for the project. This in turn meant that the staff who took on the role did not all have the necessary skills. Despite the variations in key workers' skills, the steering group had difficulty getting staff to take part in the training and none took up the offer of a mentor.

Managers noted that most key workers were not pro-active in contacting families. One attributed this to a misunderstanding between the steering group and key workers early in the project, with key workers believing that it was intended to be a reactive service. Another felt the steering group had failed to enthuse key workers and were unclear what they expected from people taking on the role. Over the course of the project, key workers were said to have given less priority to the project. This was said to mirror what was happening in the steering group who were not pro-active in supporting key workers and encouraging them to maintain regular contact with families.

The model for the key worker service in this area stated that key workers should carry out coordinated needs assessments. However, the steering group decided not to push key workers to do this. There were two reasons for this decision. First, most families involved in the project had already been assessed by the different agencies and it seemed unnecessary to undertake another assessment just so that families could have a joint care plan. Second, expecting key workers to coordinate the production of such plans was thought to be unrealistic, since many were not in a powerful enough position to take this on without there being an agreement at a higher level within their organisation. Such an agreement was never put in place.

Reflections on managing change and implementation

With hindsight, the managers felt there were a number of things the steering group should have done differently.

The steering group should have been more firmly rooted within each organisation

This would have ensured that when one person left the group someone else from within their organisation took their place.

Allocated time for the key worker role

Managers now recognised that they needed to be able to give people protected time for working with the family and attending training sessions.

A selection process for key workers

Experiences on the project also caused managers to review the recruitment process. They had accepted all volunteers for the role. However, they were now aware that key workers needed a core set of skills which many staff did not possess, suggesting that there should be some form of selection process.

Regular training and monitoring provided by a coordinator

Concerns about the skills of staff involved in the project also led managers to say that supervision for key workers needed to be built into the model. This training should have focused on the complexities of joint working, and made it clear to key workers that they were to be pro-active in liaising with families. Furthermore, key workers' progress needed to be monitored more closely so that they could be offered appropriate support.

Implementation on a smaller scale

This would have allowed managers to use their resources to monitor individual cases closely and adjust the service accordingly.

Reflections on the key worker model

Overall managers felt they had produced a very clear model and job description. Difficulties experienced in setting up a key worker service were said to be more related to the context in which they had tried to implement the model rather than the model per se. There was a firm belief that 'tinkering with the model' would not be enough to achieve a successful key worker service in their area. However, managers did suggest one adjustment to their model.

The service should be offered to families at the time of diagnosis

For the purposes of the pilot project, the steering group in Site B decided that only families who had been using services for a year or more would be eligible for a key worker. This was based on an assumption that working with these families would be easier for key workers, since they would not have to put all the services needed by the family into place. In practice, it was very difficult for key workers to penetrate and find a role within a system which was already established. When key workers contacted families they tended to say they already had everything they needed, or would ask key workers to help them access services which had already been refused. As a result, managers felt that in the future the service should be offered to families at the point of diagnosis.

Key findings

- The context into which the pilot key worker service was introduced was important. Successful implementation was reported to depend on: managers being committed to key worker services; some multi-agency working already being in place; and a steering group firmly rooted within each organisation.

- The training and skills of staff taking on the key worker role influenced the service provided. On reflection, managers suggested that staff should have gone through a selection process and been provided with training, particularly in negotiation, time-management, and assertiveness skills.

- In order for key workers to have a good understanding of their role, and the tasks they should and should *not* undertake, clear model and job description was reported to be essential.

- The ongoing support offered to key workers was found to be important. It is recommended that all key worker services have a coordinator who can take on this responsibility. Multi-agency key worker support meetings are also helpful to staff taking on the role. The need for protected time for key worker role was acknowledged by managers.

- To prevent misunderstandings about the purpose of the key worker service and to maintain enthusiasm among staff, ongoing communication between the steering group and all stakeholders was reported to be necessary.

6
Implications and recommendations

For the two sites involved, this project was, in their own words, an extremely valuable venture and learning experience. In this final chapter, we consider the implications of the findings of our evaluation of the two pilot key workers: what we learnt both in terms of our understanding of key working and, equally important, the process of setting up a key worker service. Leading on from this, we then report the very specific and practical ideas and recommendations for setting up a key worker service which were generated and developed by the two sites who worked with us on this project. Following a consideration of the limitations of this project, we conclude by considering, at a more general level, what this project can tell us about innovation and change in multi-agency settings.

Implications of the findings

In essence, by the end of the project a clear distinction had emerged between the professionals who were in contact with their pilot family at the end of the project. Some had been key workers while others were what we called 'unsuccessful' key workers. In addition, the accounts of all those families who had received a true key worker service were very positive.

From this, two fundamental questions emerge. First, what leads to a family feeling they have received a key worker service? Second, what needs to be in place to support the implementation and on-going provision of such a service? In Chapter 1, we argued that to understand any intervention or change, the approach must be one of realistic evaluation. Realistic evaluation examines the process of implementing or managing change, as well as the outcome of that change. In order to fully answer these questions, we need to draw together the accounts, gathered over the course of this project, of parents, key workers and the managers responsible for implementing the pilot services.

Understanding key worker services

From the accounts of families who had received a key worker service, we identified what we called the six key elements of key working:

- pro-active, regular contact;

- a supportive, open relationship;

- a family-centred approach;

- working across agencies;

- working with families' strengths and ways of coping;

- working for the family as opposed to working for an agency.

These were the aspects of the service that parents valued and found distinctive compared to the other forms of support they received from statutory agencies.

What was abundantly clear from the interviews with both key workers and managers, was that the ability of a professional to provide a key worker service was dependent on two key factors. First, the organisational context needed to be one in which multi-agency working was in place and there was a commitment to promote and support efforts at inter-agency working. Second, the initial and ongoing training and supervision needs of key workers needed to be identified and met.

A model of key working

These various findings can be incorporated into a model of key working which we have represented as a series of concentric circles with the disabled child and their family at the centre (see Figure 4). This model embeds key working in the foundations of a supportive organisational context - this forms the outermost ring. Parents in this study noted the importance of a key worker having the appropriate skills and qualities. These qualities are similar to those identified in other research into effective help giving and developing partnerships between parents and

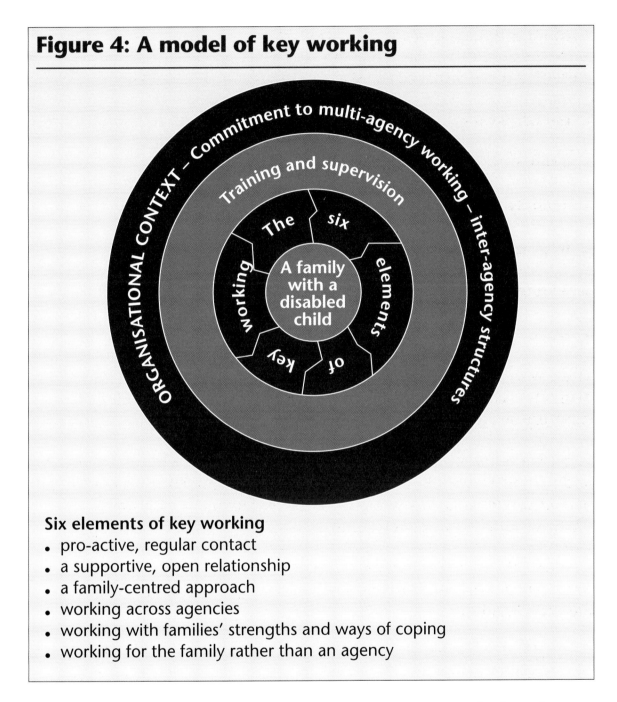

Figure 4: A model of key working

Six elements of key working
- pro-active, regular contact
- a supportive, open relationship
- a family-centred approach
- working across agencies
- working with families' strengths and ways of coping
- working for the family rather than an agency

professionals (for example, Dunst et al, 1988, 1994; Beresford et al, 1996; Dale, 1996) and include:

- basic counselling and communication skills;

- respect for parents' and children's expertise about their own lives;

- a partnership approach;

- negotiation skills;

- knowledge of disability and services provided by *all* relevant agencies (health, education, social services, housing, leisure, voluntary agencies, benefits and welfare rights).

Thus a second pre-requisite to key working - and represented by the next ring - is supervision and training. This, in itself, needs to be embedded in notions of multi-agency working, with training being offered on all agencies or organisations involved in providing services to disabled children and their families. In addition, as this project found, are the benefits of some supervision being offered in a multi-agency group context.

These two outer rings encircle the key worker ring, which we have divided into six segments to represent the six elements of key working described earlier. These segments are divided by zigzag lines as an attempt to represent the fact that the size of the segments can change. This highlights the importance of the individualistic and responsive nature of key working. Thus, while we would argue that all six elements need to be present, different elements of key working may be more important or appropriate to some families than others. Thus the 'size' of the elements - in terms of their contribution to key working with a family - can change. Finally, at the centre, is the family. This reiterates the fact that key working is for families, not for agencies - and not just for the disabled child.

Lessons to learn about planning and implementing a key worker service

Overall, different aspects of the implementation seem to have been successful in the two sites. Site A's focus on providing staff with training and supervision seems to have 'worked' in that they were successful in putting key workers in to place who, on the whole, sustained pro-active contact with families and liaised with other agencies on the families' behalf. Site B's concern with recruiting volunteers, by persuading staff that key worker services were a good thing for both themselves and families, was successful in that key workers were enthusiastic about the service and willing to stay involved, despite the difficulties they had encountered.

In order to successfully implement a key worker service, we would suggest the following aspects need to be addressed. We would also strongly recommend that more general issues around managing and implementing change in inter-agency contexts need to be taken into consideration. These are explored and addressed in our earlier report (Sloper et al, 1999).

Context and resources

- Some degree of joint working between all three key statutory agencies needs to be in place before setting up a multi-agency key worker service. While key working may well promote inter-agency working, it cannot be used to make it happen in the first place. Multi-agency planning groups, for example, can support introduction of such services at a high level within individual organisations.

- Any funding necessary for the service needs to be secured in the early stages of the implementation.

- All agencies, and departments within the relevant agencies, need to be committed to the notion of providing a multi-agency key worker service.

Planning the service

- Steering groups managing the implementation need to be firmly rooted within organisations to ensure that when one person leaves the group their place is taken by someone else within the organisation.

- All the key stakeholders need to be kept fully informed and, where appropriate, involved in planning and developing the key worker service. This applies to professionals working at all levels of the organisations involved - managers and practitioners - as well as parents. This promotes 'ownership' of the change and is less likely to result in resistance to, or sabotage of, the proposed change.

- A very clear model of a key worker service and a job description should be developed. This needs to be sensitive to the organisational and resource context in which the service will be implemented. This model needs to include provision of 'cover' key workers in the event of prolonged absence by a key worker.

- In planning the service, it is important to be aware that certain occupations or professions may constrain an individual's ability to be a key worker, such as jobs which make it difficult to leave the workplace to conduct home visits.

Supporting key working

- A coordinator, with responsibility for day-to-day management of the service, including the organisation of training and supervision is essential.

- Providing some supervision in multi-agency key worker groups is valuable.

- Key workers need to be given protected time for the role. This needs to be formally arranged, authorised and monitored to ensure that this commitment from line managers and organisations is maintained.

- Staff who take on the key worker role need to go through a selection process to ensure they have appropriate personal qualities, and their training needs are identified.

- There needs to be an acknowledgement and acceptance across all organisations involved that when a key worker is acting as an advocate for a family, they need to be independent and not constrained by any other professional or statutory responsibilities they may have.

Dealing with the specifics: ideas and suggestions

In addition to this more generic list, we have also included in this report the very specific ideas and recommendations generated by the two sites. These were developed collectively by the sites on three occasions. First at a workshop just prior to implementation of the pilot services; second, at a workshop during the implementation period; and then final revisions were made when feedback on the evaluation of the pilots had been provided. In actual fact, the 'messages' changed very little after the final revisions, the main changes being that the 'final' version carries a stronger message in terms of the need for initial and on-going commitment from all agencies and the fact that multi-agency working must already exist. The sites also became more prescriptive in terms of the need for a coordinator post and sufficient, on-going training. In addition, the importance of communication was given more emphasis - communication at a management level within and across agencies, communication within the project steering groups, communication across hierarchies within agencies, and communication with families. These 'messages from the sites' are reproduced in Box 4.

Limitations of the project

In discussing the findings, we need to acknowledge the limitations of the project and what these mean in terms of the conclusions we can draw from the research. First, in this project we undertook to implement key worker services in a very specific context: both sites were new unitary authorities and while one site lacked any formal structures for inter-agency working, there was an enthusiasm for it. Second, both sites were relatively small authorities and there is clearly a need to explore and test out this model of key working in the larger, more diverse settings. Third, neither site tested the key worker model on ethnic minority groups. Site B did assign one key worker to a family for whom English was a second language. However, the relationship between the key worker and family quickly broke down, primarily due to communication difficulties. This highlights the need for systematic piloting of key worker services with ethnic minority groups. Fourth, these were both pilot services and our evaluation of these services took place between nine and 12 months after a key worker began working with a family. We have neither been able to explore the long-term impact key working may have on families' needs and circumstances, nor its impact on key workers themselves and the organisational context in which it takes place.

Finally, given that these were pilot projects, we have been unable to observe and examine the processes and structures required to maintain and generalise a key worker service. However, it is worth noting that

Box 4: Setting up a key worker service: messages from the sites

Starting off

- Integrated multi-agency working must already exist.
- Find a 'champion' who can initiate the process.
- Ensure commitment from senior managers and maintain this commitment through regular feedback throughout.
- Involve all the relevant agencies - health commissioners and providers, education, social services, voluntary agencies.
- Keep the needs of children and families at the forefront - involve families.
- Gather basic information on numbers of disabled children and their needs.
- Identify key people who should be involved in planning the service:
  - who can make decisions and make it happen;
  - ensure representation of all relevant agencies;
  - each person should bring and maintain a positive commitment from their agency.
- Identify a steering group with representation from all agencies.
- Have parent(s) on the steering group.
- Organise time out for:
  - establishing relationships;
  - ensuring shared understanding;
  - team building;
  - planning and developing the service.
- Arrange a neutral venue and an external facilitator for this process.
- Recognise the importance of group processes.

Planning the service

- Review existing published material.
- Don't underestimate the time needed to plan and implement the service.
- Link in with, and obtain information from, other authorities who have a key worker service.
- Define the aims and principles underlying your key worker service.

- Develop and define your own local model for the service - appropriate to local needs and resources.
- Define the role of the key workers:
  - develop a job description and person specification;
  - define the boundaries of the role.
- Integrate into existing service provision.
- Issues to be addressed regarding key workers:
  - the size of the key worker service;
  - who will become key workers? - be open minded about who could be key workers;
  - who will manage, supervise and support key workers?;
  - who will provide initial and on-going training?;
  - identify who will coordinate the service;
  - ensure plans are in place to deal with leaving/sickness/disputes/difficulties.
- Issues to consider regarding families:
  - criteria for eligibility;
  - matching of key worker to family;
  - contract;
  - start/finish periods;
  - obligations/responsibilities;
  - accessibility of key worker;
  - expectations.
- Consider the wider audience - who needs to support the project? who will be affected?
- Ensure effective communication throughout.
- Develop clear action plans with defined time-scales and responsibilities.
- Be realistic about action plans - don't set them up to fail.
- Keep children and families as the prime focus.
- Record action plans and monitor progress against them.
- Consider involving an outside agency in monitoring and evaluation.

Developing and implementing the service

- Communication - share information with everyone who may be interested or affected:

- consult with families;
- consult with professionals;
- use different media - letters, newsletters, local press and radio.
- Identify key workers as soon as possible so that they have proper ownership, feel involved in the project and can be part of decision making.
- Identify training needs for steering group, key workers, coordinator.
- Develop initial training programme.
- Monitor and provide for ongoing training needs.
- Develop systems for recording the work of the service.
- Clarify systems for management and supervision of key workers.
- Clarify systems for inter-agency liaison.
- Don't underestimate the potential difficulties/constraints within and between agencies - spend time to iron these out.
- Recruit families and match key workers.
- Organise time out for reflection and further planning.
- Enjoy learning from developing the new initiative - celebrate success.

Monitoring, review and evaluation

- Decide what is going to be evaluated.
- Decide who will evaluate - internal? external?
- Decide when evaluation should take place.
- Develop consistent methods of recording.
- Monitor during regular supervision.
- Define outcomes.
- Develop a system to evaluate outcomes for families (eg, questionnaires, focus groups).

Most important priorities

- Having time out for planning.
- Making sure the service is the outcome of agreed ownership between agencies.
- Having external facilitator to point out the importance of issues of change and group process.
- In terms of evaluation, families to be involved in identifying outcomes according to their needs.

the sites involved were very clear that the way they would move forward and develop 'mainstream' key worker services would be based on the experiences of developing and implementing their pilot services.

Conclusions

This project was carried out during a period in which change and innovation was not an uncommon experience. Indeed, both sites had recently undergone the not insignificant change of becoming new unitary authorities. However, the problem with many changes (undertaken voluntarily or forced) is that while the end-product may be clear, how organisations should go about achieving such a change is very unclear and no guidance is offered.

This project - by taking an approach which was equally interested in the process of change, as well as the change itself, *and* which consulted with all the main stakeholders - has enabled us to offer our ideas both of what a key worker service should be like, and how to go about achieving one. The direct input of managers and practitioners has meant that we have been able not just to produce generic guidelines for implementing a key worker service, but also very specific and practical ideas and recommendations which, we believe, will be a valuable resource to other areas wishing to draw on the lessons learnt from this project. Finally, this project has been about key working, however, we would argue that many of the issues experienced, and in some cases overcome, during the course of this project apply to any situation where the introduction of change across agencies is trying to be achieved.

Postscript: what the sites did next...

Both sites involved in this project are committed to incorporating a key worker service as part of the support they provide to families with a disabled child. Site A plans to offer a key worker service to all families whose child has just been diagnosed as having complex needs and those families 'in transition' between child and adult services. An action plan to take this process forward has been drawn up which aims to see the service starting up during the year 2000.

Since being involved in the project, Site B has been developing an inter-agency strategy and model of service which includes a key worker service. They recognise the need to strengthen inter-agency structures before 'rolling out' a key worker service which would operate within joint children's disability teams. It is this preliminary, foundation-building, work to which Site B is first turning its attention.

References

Appleton, P., Boll, V., Everett, J.M., Kelly, A.M., Meredith, K.H. and Payne, T.G. (1997) 'Beyond child development centres: care coordination for children with disabilities', *Child: Care, Health and Development*, vol 23, no 1, pp 29-40.

Baldwin, S. and Carlisle, J. (1994) *Social support for disabled children and their families: A review of the literature*, Edinburgh: HMSO.

Beresford, B. (1994) *Positively parents: Caring for a disabled child*, London: HMSO.

Beresford, B. (1995) *Expert opinions: A survey of parents caring for a severely disabled child*, Bristol: The Policy Press.

Beresford, B., Sloper, P., Baldwin, S. and Newman, T. (1996) *What works in services for families with a disabled child?*, Barkingside: Barnardo's.

Cameron, J. and Sturge-Moore, L. (1990) *Ordinary, everyday families: Action for families and their young children with special needs, disabilities and learning difficulties*, London: Mencap.

Chamba, R., Ahmad, W., Hirst, M., Lawton, D. and Beresford, B. (1999) *On the edge: Minority ethnic families caring for a severely disabled child*, Bristol: The Policy Press.

Dale, N. (1996) *Working with families of children with special needs: Partnership and practice*, London: Routledge.

DHSS (Department of Health and Social Security) (1976) *Fit for the future: Court Committee Report on child health services*, London: HMSO.

DoH (Department of Health) (1999) *Partnership in action (new opportunities for joint working between health and social services): A discussion document*, London: DoH.

Dunst, C., Trivette, C. and Deal, A. (1988) *Enabling and empowering families: Principles and guidelines for practice*, Cambridge, MA: Brookline Books.

Dunst, C., Trivette, C. and Deal, A. (1994) *Supporting and strengthening families volume 1: Methods, strategies and practices*, Cambridge, MA: Brookline Books.

Glendinning, C. (1986) *A single door: Social work with families of disabled children*, London: Allen and Unwin.

Ovretveit, J. (1993) *Coordinating community care: Multidisciplinary teams and care management*, Milton Keynes: Open University Press.

Pawson, R. and Tilley, N. (1997) *Realistic evaluation*, London: Sage Publications.

Sloper, P. and Turner, S. (1992) 'Service needs of families of children with severe physical disability', *Child: Care, Health and Development*, vol 18, no 5, pp 259-82.

Sloper, P., Mukherjee, S., Beresford, B., Lightfoot, J. and Norris, P. (1999) *Real change not rhetoric: Putting research into practice in multi-agency services*, Bristol: The Policy Press.

Smale, G. (1996) *Mapping change and innovation*, London: HMSO.

SSI (Social Services Inspectorate)/Goodinge, S. (1998) *Inspection of services to disabled children and their families*, London: DoH.

While, A., Citrone, C. and Cornish, J. (1996) *A study of the needs and provisions for families caring for children with life-limiting incurable disorders*, London: Department of Nursing Studies, Kings College.

Appendix A: About the project: design and methods

This project involved facilitating, observing and evaluating the implementation of pilot key worker services for families with a disabled child in two local authority areas – we refer to them as 'sites' in this report. Both sites had been identified to the research team as local authorities wishing to move forward their services for disabled children and were also interested in the concept of key working. When approached by the research team, the two sites were very keen to be involved in the project.

In order to understand the context and basis of this report, this section will provide a brief overview of the project's aims and objectives, our research design and the methods we used.

Aims and objectives of the project

The aims and objectives of the project can be divided into research objectives and the objectives of the sites taking part in the project.

In terms of *research objectives*, they were as follows:

In two case sites:

i) to disseminate research findings on key workers and, working with professionals in these sites, to identify the problems and opportunities in implementing these findings;
ii) to monitor and evaluate the process of developing and implementing a pilot key worker service;
iii) to evaluate the key worker service from the point of view of families, key workers and the steering group managing implementation;
iv) to draw up guidelines for use by other local authorities about developing and implementing a key worker service;
v) at a more general level, to gain insight into the processes by which research can be put into practice more effectively.

The *sites' objectives* were as follows:

i) to develop strategies to put into place a pilot key worker service;
ii) to implement these strategies;

iii) to develop an understanding about the process of implementing multi-agency change.

The work of the project

The main way the researchers worked with the sites was through a series of joint workshops with the steering groups from the two sites held over a period of just less than two years. Each steering group consisted of representatives – managers and practitioners – from the three main statutory agencies. In one site, voluntary agencies were also represented as they were key providers in that authority.

The project began in January 1997, with initial meetings with representatives in both sites taking place in spring of that year. The first joint workshop attended by the two sites' project steering groups took place in September 1997. Development of the pilot key worker services in both sites followed that workshop, with implementation of the pilot service occurring during late spring/summer 1998. Evaluation of the outcomes of the pilot was carried out in late spring 1999.

Data gathered during the course of the project included:

i)   Material generated during the project workshops.
ii) Individual telephone interviews with professionals taking on the key worker role were carried out at the time of starting key working with a family (referred to as 'before interviews') and at the end of the pilot ('follow-up interviews'). The period over which the pilot key worker service ran in the two sites was between nine to 12 months. At the time of the second interview a 'key worker activities scale' was completed (see Appendix B).
iii) At the end of the pilot, individual interviews were conducted with parents in their homes. Parents also completed the 'key worker activities scale'.
iv) Managers who were members of the project's steering groups in the two sites were interviewed by telephone at the end of the pilot.

Appendix B: Key worker activities questionnaire

As key worker for the family, to what extent have you taken on the following tasks or roles?

Please could you rate the extent to which you have taken on the following tasks by placing a cross along each line at a point that corresponds to your view.

Advocate
Not at all ——————————————————————— Very much

Information source
Not at all ——————————————————————— Very much

Advisor
Not at all ——————————————————————— Very much

Source of emotional support
Not at all ——————————————————————— Very much

Source of practical help
Not at all ——————————————————————— Very much

Accessing new services
Not at all ——————————————————————— Very much

Service coordinator
Not at all ——————————————————————— Very much

Identifying families' needs
Not at all ——————————————————————— Very much

Formal assessment of families needs
Not at all ——————————————————————— Very much

Do you see yourself as being a key worker *primarily* for the child or for the whole family?

Child-focused   ❏
Family-focused   ❏

Appendix C: Examples of key worker services currently in operation

The named worker support service: KIDS Family Centre, Camden, London

The KIDS Family Centre is a family support centre available to all families with a child with special needs living in Camden. It was set up by KIDS, a charitable voluntary organisation.

Aims of service

To provide support, counselling, guidance and advice to parents and the whole family through regular long-term contact. Frequency of contact is negotiated individually with each family. Contact is more frequent during the period when the worker and family are getting to know each other.

Functions of service

- An advisory networking service facilitating the family's external relations.
- Assisting the family and child in dealing with their own problems and challenges around disability and special needs in the child.

Service provided to ...

Initially just families with pre-school-aged children who were using the KIDS Family Centre. However, many wanted to stay in touch with their named worker after their child started school and they no longer used the centre. This eventually led to over-demand for the service so a separate service, called the Family Project, was set up specifically to serve families of school-aged children.

Ethos

The approach of the service was to develop an 'active partnership relationship' between the named worker and the family.

Professionals providing the service

All staff working at the KIDS Family Centre, including pre-school and primary school teachers, a nursery worker, social worker, occupational and speech therapist and a clinical child psychologist.

Training
Named workers received training in child development, learning techniques and disability issues. Also training in Portage home learning methods and counselling.

Organisational issues
Because the KIDS Centre is a voluntary agency, the named workers have less power than statutory professionals in obtaining services. It also means they can be discounted and marginalised. Staff have to work hard at developing and maintaining close cooperative contact with other professionals in health, education and social services, and this is time-consuming.

Other comments
The KIDS centre is a voluntary agency, and parents value the impartiality and independence of their named worker.

Source and further information
Dale (1996).

Care coordination project: Wrexham

Aims of service
To provide a single named person to coordinate care and education for a disabled child and his/her family.

Functions of service
- To provide a structure assessment of the whole family's needs.
- To provide a care plan (incorporating a school transition plan).
- To offer continuity of availability for parents throughout the period of transition to nursery school.
- Coordinating case reviews.

Service provided to ...
Children in transition to nursery school. The service was subsequently extended, in modified forms, to other populations.

Ethos
The care coordinator was seen as a means of bridging agencies and bridging the pre-school to nursery transition. The care coordinator was also seen as a means of matching need to service.

Professionals providing the service
Professionals from a number of services including clinical medical officers, social workers, and community nurses.

Training
Initial and continued training was seen as vital, especially listening, coordination, assessment and care planning skills. They also note the importance of training administrative staff.

Organisational issues
The project stresses the importance of the care coordinator being able to communicate freely across services within a "supportive, client-focused, interagency context". This requires a full commitment from senior professionals and senior managers to create that context for front-line staff. A full-time inter-agency development officer is reported to have

been "crucial in maintaining progress in genuine local strategic change". Support and supervision of care coordinators are seen as important.

Other comments

Unlike the other examples, this project was systematically based on principles of care coordination and care management laid down in various policy documents and academic literature. They would probably disagree that they were providing a key worker service, arguing that key workers are service specific (Ovretveit, 1993).

Source and further information

Appleton et al (1997).

Dr P. Appleton, School of Psychology, University of Wales, Bangor, Gwynedd LL57 2DG.

Peter Lund, Development Officer, Personal Services Directorate, Wrexham County Borough, Lambpit Street, PO Box 1286, Wrexham LL11 1WG.

The One Hundred Hours key worker model

One Hundred Hours is a voluntary agency which provides a key worker to families as soon as possible after diagnosis or the birth of a child with multiple disabilities.

Aims

To be a stopgap service for families until statutory support services are in place, offering a high level of contact and support through, at least, weekly visits. The service is time-limited to around a hundred hours by which time it is hoped that statutory services are ready to take over.

Functions

- To give emotional support.
- To provide information - both about the child's condition and support services.
- To help and support parents as they access statutory support services. This might involve liaison with professionals, organising/attending case conferences etc.
- To provide a 'parent programme'. This is a programme of activities and therapies drawing on physiotherapy, speech therapy and teaching skills which is given to parents to use at home to promote the child's well-being and development.

Ethos

There is no fixed formula for the type of service provided. The family decides the key worker's role and establishes priorities.

Professionals providing the service

A number of workers from various disciplines are key workers for One Hundred Hours. They do not assume their typical role (eg, physiotherapist, teacher) when acting as a key worker. They draw on skills from a number of professions when devising the parent programme.

Training

Training in counselling and welfare services is provided. There is also a considerable amount of 'skill sharing'.

Organisational issues

Referrals are taken from hospitals in the region, or families can self-refer. Take up of the service by different hospitals varies enormously, depending largely perhaps on differing perceptions of families' needs. The effectiveness of the key worker is, to some extent, dependent on the degree to which professionals in the statutory agencies respect and acknowledge the key worker's role and position.

Source and further information

Peter Limbrick, One Hundred Hours, Dobroyd Castle, Todmorden, West Yorkshire OL14 7JJ.

Appendix D: Further demographic and organisational information about the sites

Site A – North East Lincolnshire
Demographic factors
North East Lincolnshire is situated on the south eastern side of the Humber Estuary on the east coast of England. It covers 192 square kilometres and is surrounded on three sides by water. North East Lincolnshire has a population of approximately 160,000, with minority ethnic groups making up 1% of the population. Forty thousand people are under the age of 18. The major centres of population (accounting for more than 80% of the authority's population) are Grimsby and Cleethorpes. In 1991, there were an estimated 745 children under the age of 16 reported to have some form of limiting long-term illness, handicap or condition, representing 2% of the total child population of that age.

On many social and economic indicators North East Lincolnshire displays considerable social need. In October 1996, there was an unemployment rate of 9.3% which is higher than the national average of 7%. In some areas, this rises to 33%. There are pockets of low income and deprivation. On average, 21% of households were living in poverty, compared to the national average of 19%. But this masks considerable differences within the authority, as scores range from 11% to 32% of households in poverty in different parts of the authority.

Organisational context
North East Lincolnshire is one of the new unitary authorities. The administrative area of North East Lincolnshire was created in March 1995 and officially came into force in April 1996. A co-terminus, combined acute and community health trust – North East Lincolnshire NHS Trust – was formed in 1993. At the beginning of the project the voluntary sector (Barnardo's) was becoming increasingly involved in the provision of services for disabled children and their families.

Overall, some degree of joint working was in place at the start of this project and this increased over the period of our involvement with this site. In 1996, the council carried out a strategic review of services to disabled children. A multi-disciplinary working group was set up and was chaired independently by Barnardo's. Some members of the project's steering group sat on this working group. After this review the multi-disciplinary working group developed the following policy:

- an organisational commitment to working corporately;

- the development of inter-agency working and sharing of experience;

- ensure accessibility of service provision;

- to assess individual needs, plan reviews and monitor all services provision to children with disabilities and their families.

Following the review of services, the service planning group set up a number of development plans for disabled children. At the beginning of the project, managers from the area were in process of setting up a resource centre for disabled children and their families, staffed by a multi-agency group, including Barnardo's. This centre opened in early summer 1998. The centre aims to make life easier for families by providing clear information, giving a clear point of entry to services, coordinating assessment of need and possible delivery, and developing new ways of working within existing resources.

Site B – Middlesbrough
Demographic factors
Middlesbrough is a large town in the north east of England with a population of approximately 146,000. A total of 4.4% of the population describe themselves as belonging to a minority ethnic group. Forty-three thousand people in Middlesbrough are under the age of 19. In 1997, it was estimated that more than 3% of 0- to 15-year-olds had a health or disability problem. Higher than national average health and disability problems occur in 19 out of Middlesbrough's 25 wards.

Middlesbrough is ranked as one of the most disadvantaged non-metropolitan towns in England. There are higher than average levels of unemployment, lone parenthood, health/disability problems, and standard mortality rates. During 1996-97, over 1,200 children from the town were referred to social services for child protection services. Another 4,250 were referred as children in need.

Organisational context

Middlesbrough is a 'new' unitary authority, also coming into operation in April 1996. It has separate community and acute health trusts (South Tees Acute Hospitals NHS Trust and South Tees Community and Mental Health NHS Trust) which are not coterminus with the local authority.

At the start of the project, managers from the three key statutory agencies were not meeting on a regular basis. Joint working structures were not in place and there was no joint funding of services for disabled children and their families. It was clear from their Children's Services Plan (CSP) that joint working/commissioning was something on which Middlesbrough was wanting to move forward. Within their CSP are these two objectives:

- the development of coordinated services for children with special needs, with a singular assessment and management function;

- joint commissioning, between social services, the health authority and education, of specialist services for children with special needs.

Appendix E: Key worker job decriptions

Site A: job description

Job purpose

Make life easier for parents
Make life easier for families
First contact for families/agencies
Early/earliest possible intervention/involvement
Empowering families – not 'dependency'
Improve multi-agency working
Enable multi-agency working
Developing parents' coping mechanisms
Ensuring things get done – at reviews – preventing 'drift'
Support/counselling
Knowledge of statutory requirements for children with disabilities

Skills

Communication – not imposing own values
Listening
Building relationships – exploring/knowing options – to inform choices
Developing 'people skills'
Negotiating skills
Non-judgemental

Background experience

Knowledge/involvement with children with disability
Working knowledge of 'multi-agency'

Personality/style

Good relationship skills
Empathy

Site B: job description
Job title: Key Worker for families and children with disabilities
Responsible to: Individual service manager, ie status quo
Mentor: Designated member of the Project Steering Group

Definition of key worker in this pilot study
A named professional who will:

- coordinate and/or facilitate assessments and reviews being undertaken by health, social services and education in respect of a child with disabilities;
- coordinate the production of a single care plan which sets out how the assessed educational, health and social care needs of the child will be met;
- act as a first point of contact for the parent/carer/child seeking advice, information, guidance, support and assistance;
- facilitate communication between agencies and the parent/carer/child.

Key result areas
1. Parents/carers and children will clearly identify and have confidence in the key worker as the professional who can support them and coordinate their holistic needs.
2. Other professionals in all agencies will support the key worker to ensure effective coordinated care for the child and family.
3. Production of a single care plan for the child and family involving all agencies and reviewed systematically.

Specific responsibilities
1. Ensure that the family/carer/child understands the role of the key worker and agree together how and when the key worker can be contacted.
2. Advise all the other professionals and agencies working with the child and family of the key worker role and contact arrangements.
3. Coordinate the production of a written care plan for the child and family, indicating assessed needs, outcomes and target dates for achievement and services to be provided.

4. Review the care statement regularly (every four to six months) with the family. Take action as necessary.

5. Coordinate the review of the care statement at least annually with all professionals and the family/child to monitor achievement of the outcomes and maintain effective support to the child. Ensure that agreed revisions to the care statement are implemented.

6. Identify gaps in service needed to meet short-term needs of the child and family to individual service manager to facilitate forward planning.

7. Familiarise themselves with the range of services available from all agencies and voluntary bodies to ensure the child and family receive appropriate support and input. Involve other agencies and professionals as appropriate.

8. With agreement, distribute a copy of the care statement to other agencies and professionals involved with the family's needs (eg GP and Primary Health Care Team).

9. Act as a point of contact for other agencies and professionals who need information and advice about the child's and family's needs.

10. During the pilot project:
   - work with the Steering Group and reviewers from the Social Policy Research Unit, University of York, to assess and monitor progress of the pilot and evaluate the benefits and operation of the key worker project;
   - participate in the training programmes;
   - take part in monthly support group meetings.

I.D. No.   1361263

UNIVERSITY of BRADFORD

2 8 MAR 2001

ACCESSION No. 0343027332

CLASS No. D 306, 278 MUK

LOCATION